Chapter 1: The O

I was a normal, healthy person who was focused on being fairly fit and strong. Martial arts, yoga, cycling, and daily walks along the beach were all part of my lifestyle. At the same time, I was not a complete fitness fanatic. I enjoyed a drink now and then, snacks, and the occasional takeaway. But overall, I was active, disciplined, and healthy.

Then, suddenly and without warning, everything changed. Out of the blue, I was struck by a rare disease. At first, I thought it was something minor, maybe fatigue or overexertion, but the symptoms quickly grew worse. I went to a doctor, hoping for answers and relief. Instead, I was given some medicines and told to come back in five days.

Those five days felt like a lifetime. The medication brought no improvement. In fact, I felt progressively worse with each passing day. My balance began to fail me, my eyesight was no longer sharp, and a constant tingling sensation spread through my feet. The most alarming moment came when I realised I could no longer even pass urine.

That was when my loyal employee Shankar, along with my former employee Ravi who had a taxi, rushed me to a hospital in Mapusa. Their quick action spared me from further complications. I was deeply grateful to them, though at that moment, gratitude was mixed with confusion and fear. I had no idea what was happening to me, only that my body was no longer under my control.

Chapter 2: The First Symptoms

At the hospital in Mapusa, the doctors acted quickly. They put a catheter in me and started me on heavy medication. I was kept in the ICU for a couple of nights before being shifted to a room. I felt a small sense of relief, believing that now I was under professional care, answers would surely come.

But that relief did not last. For five long days I was tested, observed, and medicated, yet no clear diagnosis emerged. My condition continued to worsen. I still could not pass urine without the catheter, my balance was gone, my eyesight blurred, and the tingling sensation in my feet persisted like an electric current running through me.

On the fifth day, to my shock, the doctors discharged me. No explanation, no treatment plan, just a polite but firm instruction to go home. I remember the feeling vividly—confusion, disbelief, and a rising fear. I had walked into the hospital desperate for help, and I was leaving weaker, more helpless, and with no answers.

At home, the situation weighed heavily on both me and my wife, Heidi. She tried to stay strong for me, but I could see the anxiety in her eyes. Shankar and Ravi, too, could only watch as my condition deteriorated further. My independence was slipping away from me day by day.

It was one of the lowest points of my journey. To be so unwell, yet without a name for the illness, left me feeling trapped in a nightmare. I kept asking myself: *What is wrong with me? Why can no one tell me?*

What I did not know then was that the answer—and the real turning point—was waiting for me just next door.

Chapter 3: The Wrong Turns

Being discharged from the hospital after only five days felt like being abandoned in the middle of a storm. I had walked in desperate for answers, but I left with none. The catheter remained, my legs felt heavy and unreliable, my eyesight was blurred, and the tingling in my feet was as strong as ever.

Back at home, life was no easier. The relief of being away from the hospital walls was quickly replaced by a deep sense of helplessness. I had always been independent, a man who valued discipline and physical fitness. Now, I needed help even for the smallest things. Sitting, standing, walking, even turning in bed felt like monumental tasks.

Heidi tried her best to keep things normal. She would talk to me, reassure me, and encourage me, but I could see the fear in her eyes. She had never seen me so weak. Shankar hovered around quietly, always ready to lend a hand, always alert to my needs. Their presence was comforting, but it also highlighted how much I had changed. I was no longer the strong and capable person they had known.

I felt trapped, as though I was going around in circles, searching for answers but ending up right where I started—lost, tired, and without direction. The frustration gnawed at me day and night. I kept thinking: *Why can't the doctors figure this out?*

How can they send me home like this?

My world had shrunk to the four walls of my room. The activities that once defined me—martial arts, yoga, cycling, and long walks on the beach—were now out of reach. It was as though someone had pressed pause on my life, leaving me suspended in uncertainty.

I didn't know it then, but hope was about to appear in the most unexpected way. After all the wrong turns, the right path was waiting for me just next door.

Chapter 4: Help Next Door

One evening my wife, Heidi, came to tell me that she happened to be in our garden area when she met Dr. Dattaraj Nachinolkar on his way back from work. He lived right next door to us. Dr. Datta, as we called him, is a well-renowned Orthopedic Surgeon in Goa. During their conversation, he asked about me, and Heidi told him about my recent hospitalisation and how my condition was still not improving.

Without hesitation, Dr. Datta said that he would check me. When he examined me, he immediately told me that I needed to be admitted to the hospital again. He also asked why I had not gone to him in the first place. I admitted that I had been reluctant to bother him, since he was an Orthopedic Surgeon and I thought my illness would not fall under his speciality. He reassured me kindly but firmly that he could help me, and that there was no question of being a bother—after all, he was not just a doctor, but also my neighbour.

What an enormous relief I felt that day! After going all around the block, searching for answers and finding none, the solution was right there next door. For the first time in weeks, I felt a sense of hope return.

Soon after, I was admitted to Redkar Hospital in Goa. There I underwent a battery of tests—neurological, physiological, and even psychiatric evaluations to rule out psychological issues. It was exhausting, but at least there was now a clear sense of direction.

Dr. Sagar Redkar took charge of my case. After carefully reviewing everything, the first diagnosis given was **Demyelinating Polyneuropathy**. Later, after further study and consultation, this was changed to **Guillain-Barré Syndrome (GBS)**.

Hearing the name of the disease for the first time was both frightening and relieving. Frightening, because I had never heard of GBS before and didn't know what it meant. Relieving, because at last, there was a name for what was happening to me. It was no longer a mystery—it was something real, something known, something I could now begin to fight.

Chapter 5: A Year in the Hospital

With the diagnosis of Guillain-Barré Syndrome confirmed, I began what turned out to be a year-long stay in the hospital. Nothing in my life had prepared me for it. Having been an active person, it was hard for me to accept being bedridden twenty-four hours a day.

My days quickly fell into a routine. I would be woken at 5:00 a.m., given a sponge bath, and changed into fresh clothes. Breakfast would follow, and later the doctors would come on their rounds. That was, more or less, my day—every day. It was monotonous, repetitive, and for someone like me, who was used to movement, discipline, and activity, it felt like a prison.

The days were long. I was not a fan of television, and with my eyesight not at its best, reading—the one pastime I loved—was almost impossible. Books, especially non-fiction, had always been my companions, and being cut off from them made me feel even more isolated.

Yet, despite the monotony and the frustration, I was never without gratitude. I owed my survival to Dr. Dattaraj, Dr. Redkar, the nurses and staff, my wife Heidi, and Shankar. Their dedication, care, and loyalty carried me through the darkest days of that year. I might have been confined to a bed, but I was not fighting alone.

Chapter 6: Legless on the Treadmill

After months of being bedridden, a spark of hope arrived—the physiotherapist booked me for my very first session. I was thrilled. At last, I thought, I would be active again. Even the smallest movement felt like it would be a victory after being confined to bed for so long.

On the appointed day, the staff arrived at my room with a stretcher and a device that looked like a small crane. They strapped me into a harness attached to the crane-like device and wheeled me into the physiotherapy room. There, they positioned me in front of a treadmill and instructed me to hold the bars tightly.

When the treadmill started, I realised the harness was supporting much of my weight.

My legs were moving, but I wasn't truly walking. Determined, I asked them to lower me so that my feet could take my full weight. The moment they did, I had a shocking realisation—I was legless.

Back in the UK, I used to hear friends say after a wild weekend, "Mate, I was legless on Saturday night!" At the time, I laughed, not really understanding what they meant. Now I understood in the most sobering way possible. For them, "legless" meant being drunk and stumbling, unable to control their legs. For me, it was the devastating truth that I had no sensation from the waist down. My feet touched the treadmill, but they gave me no feedback. My brain and body were no longer connected.

The physiotherapy team quickly raised me back up into the harness, and the machine carried on moving my legs. But the shock of that moment stayed with me. I had gone in excited, thinking I would walk again, but I came away humbled by the reality of how far I still had to go.

And yet, in that difficult moment, I made a silent promise to myself: I would not give up. If my legs would not obey me now, then I would fight every day until they did. The road ahead was going to be long and painful, but this was my first step—quite literally—on the path back to life.

Chapter 7: The Nightmares

As if the physical struggles were not enough, the nights often became their own kind of torture. My body was weak, but my mind, restless and overactive, conjured fears that invaded my sleep.

On some nights, I had nightmares so vivid and terrifying that they shook me to my core. I would wake up drenched in sweat, my heart pounding, unsure for a moment whether I was still dreaming or awake. The images were often about being trapped—locked in a body that refused to respond, falling into darkness with no way to stop myself, or trying to call out but finding no voice. They mirrored my real-life experience of paralysis, magnified into terrifying visions.

After a few nights of this torment, I could not bear it anymore. I asked to see a doctor, desperate for relief. That was when Dr. Pallavi, the resident psychiatrist, came to see me. She sat by my bed and listened patiently as I described the nightmares in detail. After a long, thoughtful conversation, she explained that the heavy doses of medicines I was on could very well be the cause of these disturbing dreams. She decided to adjust my treatment.

Her intuition was correct. Within days of changing the medication, the nightmares stopped. I was able to sleep peacefully through the night again. In fact, the new medicine worked so well that I often found myself napping during the day as well. For the first time in a long while, I experienced true rest.

Sleep became one of my greatest healers. It restored not only my body but also my spirit. After months of being battered by fear and uncertainty, the simple gift of uninterrupted sleep felt like a blessing.

Still, the days remained long and monotonous. Being cut off from books was a deep frustration, leaving me with too many hours of emptiness. But the absence of nightmares brought me a kind of peace, and that peace gave me the strength to carry on.

Chapter 8: Discharge Day

At last, the day came when I was to be discharged from the hospital. After being in for approximately one year, it almost felt unreal to hear those words: *You can go home.* I had grown so accustomed to the hospital routine—the doctors' visits, the nurses' care, the silence of my private room—that the thought of leaving felt like stepping into another world.

The first wave of emotion was pure joy. I was going home. The idea of being back with my wife, Heidi, with our little cat, and with the loyal staff who had stood by us, filled me with excitement. I longed for the familiar sounds, smells, and comforts of home. That first night back truly was magical. Sleeping in my own bed, seeing my surroundings again, and feeling the warmth of family around me—it was a moment of celebration.

But that initial euphoria did not last long. Very quickly, the reality set in. The hospital might have discharged me, but GBS had not let me go. Everyday tasks that once seemed effortless—standing up, walking a few steps, bathing—were now challenges that demanded every ounce of strength. I realised that while the hospital stay had been one battle, recovery at home would be another, longer war.

The road ahead looked daunting, but I reminded myself of one thing: I had always carried a positive attitude. That attitude had helped me endure the long days in the hospital, and it would help me again now. Dr. Dattaraj himself remarked that my spirit and positivity were aiding my recovery. His words stayed with me, giving me renewed courage.

I also had my support system. Heidi was my rock, caring for me with endless patience. Our little cat, with its playful presence, lifted my spirits when I felt low. And Shankar, devoted and dependable, stood by me like a faithful soldier. Together, they created a circle of care around me that made even the hardest days bearable.

Discharge day was not the end of my story with GBS. It was the beginning of a new phase—one where the setting changed, but the struggle continued. Still, as I crossed the threshold of my home that day, I carried with me something stronger than fear: hope. And with hope, I knew that step by step, no matter how slowly, I would find my way back.

Chapter 9: Walking Again

Coming home after a year in hospital was like being reborn into a different life. The comfort of my own surroundings gave me strength, but the reality of how much I had lost quickly became clear. Something as simple as walking from one room to another now felt like climbing a mountain. My legs trembled, my balance was gone, and I would sweat heavily after only a few steps.

But I refused to give up. I began slowly, holding onto the walls for support. Five steps one day, six the next. Progress was painfully slow, but it was progress. Heidi encouraged me constantly, and Shankar stayed by my side like a faithful shadow. With his steady hand, I soon managed to step outside and walk short distances around the patio. Feeling the fresh air and the sun on my face gave me a joy I had never known before. In time, I even managed to walk around the block with the help of my walking stick,

Shankar at my side, ready to catch me if I faltered.

Recovery was not just about walking. It was also about reconnecting with the practices that had shaped me before my illness. I returned to martial arts in the only way I could—through Wing Chun. I practiced **Siu Lim Tao**, the first form of Wing Chun, which is performed in a static position. Though my body was weak, those slow, deliberate movements gave me confidence. Each posture reminded me of the discipline and strength that still lived within me, even if my body had changed.

Yoga, too, called me back. One day, I decided to attempt **Surya Namaskar**—the Sun Salutation. It had always been a favorite practice of mine, a complete flow that stretched and strengthened the whole body. I began carefully, moving through the familiar poses, but when it came time to stretch backward, I lost my balance and came crashing down onto a bedside table. Fortunately, I was not badly hurt, but the fall shook me. For a few days, I rested, gathering myself again.

That fall taught me an important lesson. Recovery would not be a straight line. There would be setbacks, stumbles, and moments of discouragement. But as I told myself then, the important thing was not perfection—it was persistence. After resting, I resumed my practice, this time with more caution and respect for my limits.

Walking again was more than physical progress. It was about

reclaiming independence, rebuilding confidence, and rediscovering joy in the smallest of actions. Each step, however shaky, reminded me that I was alive, healing, and still capable of fighting my way back.

Chapter 10: Meditation as Medicine

As my body fought its slow battle to recover, my mind also needed healing. Being confined for so long forced me to sit with myself, and in that stillness, meditation became both a refuge and a tool in my fight against GBS.

I had first been introduced to **Transcendental Meditation (TM)** many years earlier, long before illness touched my life. Guru Kamalaji, a friend of my father, had organised a three-day course. Each evening, I would take a cab across the city, eager but also curious about what meditation really was. The sessions began with simple explanations—how to sit, how to breathe, how to gently quiet the mind. On the final day, she gave each of us a **guru mantra**—a secret Sanskrit word, never to be revealed—that would serve as the heart of our practice. I remember feeling both intrigued and humbled. Could the repetition of a single word really transform the mind?

In the years that followed, I practiced TM whenever I could. There were times in London, during stressful workdays, when I would close my eyes and meditate quietly in a corner. It gave me clarity, steadiness, and focus. In moments of personal struggle, I often found that meditation carried me through with calm when nothing else could. I never thought then how crucial this practice would become for me later.

Now, in the middle of my illness, I returned to that mantra with renewed dedication. I would prop myself up on pillows so my back was straight, close my eyes, and silently repeat the mantra in my mind. Slowly, the chatter of my thoughts would fade. There would be moments, sometimes just a few seconds, when everything dissolved—no "I," no "me," no ego. Just stillness. In those moments, all my problems seemed to disappear.

Meditation gave me peace at night when sleep felt impossible, and calm during the day when boredom pressed heavily on me. After twenty minutes of practice, I felt refreshed, lighter, and often ready to face physiotherapy or walking practice with more determination. It also brought deep, restorative sleep, like a baby drifting into dreams.

The beauty of meditation is that it does not demand belief,

debate, or doctrine. It is not about words—it is about experience. And my experience was profound. While religion had often left me with questions, meditation gave me something more valuable: silence. That silence, paradoxically, was full of answers.

Meditation became one of my strongest medicines. It quietened my fears, steadied my emotions, and reminded me that healing was not only about my body—it was about my spirit too. Each time I sat in stillness, I felt connected to something beyond myself. That connection gave me the strength to continue, one day at a time.

Chapter 11: Breathing Life Back

Alongside meditation, I turned to the ancient practice of **pranayama**—the science of breath in yoga. Years before, I had studied these techniques at The Yoga Institute in Mumbai, and they had always fascinated me. Now, in the quiet of my recovery, they became one of my most powerful tools for healing.

I began with **Anulom Vilom**, or alternate nostril breathing. According to yoga teachings, the breath from the right nostril energises the left hemisphere of the brain, while the breath from the left nostril energises the right hemisphere. Balancing the two creates harmony, not only in the brain but throughout the body. Sitting quietly, focusing on each breath, I could feel my nervous system calming down, as if my very circuits were being slowly repaired.

Then came **Kapalbhati**, the "skull-shining breath." With each sharp exhalation, I imagined I was expelling not only air but also weakness, toxins, and negativity. After a session of Kapalbhati, my body felt lighter, my mind clearer, and my energy stronger. It was as though the breath itself was cleansing me from within.

I continued practising Anulom Vilom and other techniques, each one providing me with a slightly different benefit. Together, they taught me that healing was not only about muscle strength or nerve recovery—it was about prana, the life force itself. Every conscious breath was a way of filling myself with energy and hope.

The discipline of pranayama gave structure to my days. Each session felt like a promise to myself: that I was actively fighting back, that I was not giving in. And slowly, I began to notice changes. My breathing became deeper, my mind calmer, and my body more responsive to the small exercises I attempted each day.

I often thought back to my yoga teachers, **Sujit Sir and Devi Madam**, whose guidance had given me the foundation to use yoga as a tool for healing. Their voices and teachings echoed in my mind as I practiced, reminding me to stay steady and patient. Combined with the knowledge I had gained from martial arts and meditation, pranayama gave me a holistic system that supported me when modern medicine alone could not.

Yoga, martial arts, meditation, and pranayama were not just

activities anymore. They became my survival kit. Each breath, each movement, each moment of silence was a weapon in my battle against GBS. With every breath, I was not just inhaling oxygen—I was breathing life back into myself.

Chapter 12: Cycling Back to Strength

As my strength slowly began to return, I began to crave the activities that had once given me joy. Walking was my first milestone, but I wanted to go further. That was when cycling re-entered my life—not just as exercise, but as a symbol of freedom.

I remembered reading an inspiring story about the founder of **Raleigh Bicycles** in Nottingham, England. This man had been gravely ill, and doctors had given him only six months to live. Instead of surrendering, he decided to fight back by cycling. Over those six months, he cycled extensively. By the end of it, instead of dying, he found that his health and strength had improved dramatically. That transformation inspired him to start the Raleigh Bicycle Company, which went on to become one of the most famous bicycle manufacturers in the world.

I have had the pleasure of visiting Nottingham on a few occasions, but sadly they were all work-related, and I never had the chance to visit the Raleigh Company—if it is still around. Still, that story stayed with me, and when I thought of cycling, it filled me with determination.

So when I became a bit better, I decided to start cycling again. It was not easy. My balance was shaky, and right turns were especially difficult. On one occasion I fell, and on another I nearly lost control. But fall or no fall, I refused to give up. Each time I got back on the bicycle and tried again. The wind in my face, the rhythm of pedalling, the sense of forward motion—it reminded me of who I had been before GBS, and who I still could be.

Even my doctor encouraged me. He advised me to cycle at least twice a week, saying that it would strengthen my legs and improve my stamina. Unlike walking, cycling did not make me sweat excessively, and I found that I could go farther without tiring as quickly.

Cycling became more than just exercise. It was therapy, motivation, and freedom rolled into one. Every ride carried me not only forward on the road but also forward in my recovery. The bicycle became my teacher, showing me that perseverance, balance, and movement—however difficult—were the keys to life after GBS.

Chapter 13: Acceptance & Reflection

During the long months of recovery, I found myself reflecting deeply on life. Being confined to bed or limited in movement gave me endless hours to think. Again and again, one question kept rising in my mind: *Why did this happen to me?*

I had always tried to stay fit. I practiced martial arts, yoga, and meditation. I cycled and walked daily. Was this the result of some bad karma? Or was it simply one of life's unpredictable turns? These questions weighed heavily on me at first. But in time, I came to realise that the only way forward was acceptance.

Acceptance did not mean giving up. It meant recognising my reality and choosing to work with it, rather than against it. I had to accept that my body had changed, that my daily life was disrupted, and that recovery would take time. Only by accepting these truths could I find the strength to move ahead.

In the dojo of life, as in martial arts training, we are faced with both techniques we enjoy and techniques we dislike. Some are easy, others are difficult. But a true martial artist must learn them all. Life is the same. We cannot choose only the pleasant experiences; we must also face the painful ones. GBS became one of those difficult lessons, teaching me patience, humility, and resilience.

Another realisation that came to me during this time was the importance of mindfulness. Looking back, I realised that in the good times, I had not always been mindful. I practiced martial arts, meditation, and yoga, and I read books on philosophy and self-improvement, but I was not always grateful for the simple fact of being healthy. It is strange how often we realise the value of something only after it is gone.

My reflections also led me to think about spirituality and the idea of God. All my life, I had heard people describe God as loving, powerful, and forgiving. But if God was truly all-loving, why was there so much suffering in the world? Why war, disease, and injustice? And why always "He"? Why not "She" or "It"? These questions left me confused, and I found no clear answers.

What I did know, however, was that I experienced something truly spiritual during meditation. In those moments of silence, when the mind dissolved and there was no "I" or "ego," I felt connected to something beyond myself. Perhaps that is what people mean when they speak of God. For me, it was not a figure or an image, but an experience.

Meditation gave me peace, and with it came gratitude. Gratitude for Heidi, who stood by me through everything. Gratitude for Shankar, whose loyalty never wavered. Gratitude for my doctors, Dr. Dattaraj and Dr. Redkar, and for the nurses and staff who cared for me. Gratitude even for the illness itself, because it taught me to see life differently.

Acceptance and reflection became as important to my

healing as medicine and physiotherapy. They reminded me that while I could not control everything, I could control how I responded. And I chose to respond with strength, gratitude, and a renewed appreciation for life.

Chapter 14: Conclusion — Yin, Yang, and Life Lessons

Looking back on my journey with Guillain-Barré Syndrome, I see it not only as a medical battle but also as one of life's greatest teachers. I had not been prepared for it, but when it came, it reshaped me—body, mind, and spirit. What once seemed like a curse slowly revealed itself as a lesson. Life is fragile, yet it is also the greatest gift we have.

Before GBS, I had taken many things for granted. I was strong, active, and full of confidence. Walking, standing, even taking a shower felt effortless. Only when those abilities were stripped away did I truly realise how precious they were. Through GBS, I learned humility. I learned gratitude. I learned that every step, every breath, every small act of independence is worth celebrating.

Yoga played a vital role in my healing. **Surya Namaskar**, the Sun Salutation, once again became a favourite practice. It burned away laziness, awakened my body, and reminded me of the rhythm of life. **Kapalbhati** and **Anulom Vilom** pranayama helped balance my mind and body, restoring energy when I felt depleted. Listening to bhajans during my yoga practice added a spiritual depth that made each session feel like prayer. Yoga taught me that healing is not only physical—it is also mental, emotional, and spiritual.

My martial arts background also gave me strength. Years earlier, when I trained in Shaolin Kung Fu with Sifu Bob Stannells in London, I learned discipline, focus, and resilience. I still remember attending a show by Shaolin monks at the Docklands Arena, where they spoke of **Bodhidharma**, the Indian monk who brought meditation and martial arts to China. He had noticed monks falling asleep during meditation, so he introduced exercises to keep them awake and strong. That story stayed with me, and I understood its truth during my own battle. Meditation and movement are not opposites—together they create balance.

This balance is what I now think of as **yin and yang**. From yoga, I drew the yin energy—soft, healing, inward. From martial arts, I drew the yang energy—strength, power, outward force. Together, they created harmony, a wholeness that gave me resilience. Healing came not from one thing alone, but from the union of many: medicine, yoga, martial arts, meditation, love, and discipline.

Perhaps the greatest lesson of all was the importance of **discipline**. Discipline is the quiet force behind success, whether in recovery or in life. Small acts—throwing rubbish in a bin, maintaining a routine, keeping promises to myself—built a foundation of strength. Just as great achievers in the world have credited discipline for their success, I too found it to be my guiding principle. Discipline, more than anything else, kept me moving forward when I felt like giving up.

The takeaway from this experience is simple yet profound: never take life for granted. **Stay alert in the present moment, be grateful for everything at all times, and try to be the best person you can be.**

GBS was the toughest challenge of my life, but it also gave me the deepest lessons. I emerged not the same man I was before—but perhaps a better one. And for that, strangely enough, I am grateful.

📖 Title Page

My Experience with Guillain-Barré Syndrome

Lessons in Strength, Healing, and Acceptance

By **Jimi G**

📖 Table of Contents

- Preface
- Chapter 1: The Onset of Illness
- Chapter 2: The First Symptoms
- Chapter 3: The Wrong Turns
- Chapter 4: Help Next Door
- Chapter 5: A Year in the Hospital
- Chapter 6: Legless on the Treadmill
- Chapter 7: The Nightmares

- Chapter 8: Discharge Day
- Chapter 9: Walking Again
- Chapter 10: Meditation as Medicine
- Chapter 11: Breathing Life Back
- Chapter 12: Cycling Back to Strength
- Chapter 13: Acceptance & Reflection
- Chapter 14: Conclusion — Yin, Yang, and Life Lessons
- The End
- Blurb

Printed in Dunstable, United Kingdom